Shape up
your bum

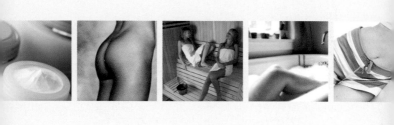

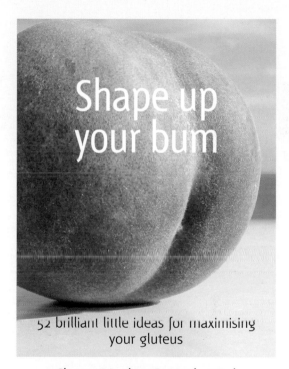

Shape up
your bum

52 brilliant little ideas for maximising
your gluteus

Cherry Maslen & Linda Bird

brilliantideas

CAREFUL NOW

Follow the tips in this book and you should find that your bottom gradually becomes more toned and pert. Don't expect miracles – perfection takes time. Before undertaking a new diet or excercise regime it's a good idea to speak to your doctor, and if you're currently taking any medication speak to her before taking any herbs or nutritional supplements.
We hope you get the curves you deserve.

Infinite Ideas would like to thank Linda Bird, Eve Cameron, Kate Cook, Helena Frith Powell, Cherry Maslen and Steve Shipside for their contributions to this book.

First published in 2007 by
The Infinite Ideas Company Limited
36 St Giles
Oxford, OX1 3LD
United Kingdom
www.infideas.com

A CIP catalogue record for this book is available from the British Library

ISBN 978-1-905940-02-8

Brand and product names are trademarks or registered trademarks of their respective owners.

Designed and typeset by Baseline Arts Ltd, Oxford
Printed in Singapore

Brilliant ideas

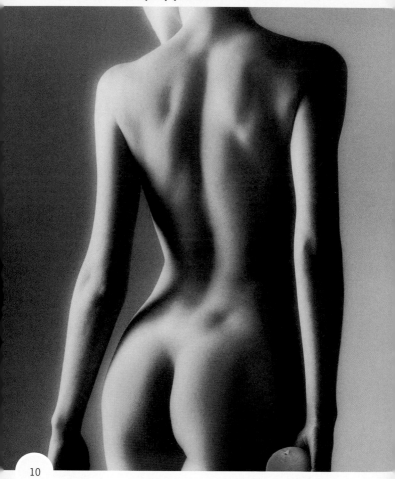

Introduction

This probably isn't the first book you've
picked up in your quest for posterior
perfection. Perhaps you've been struggling
with cellulite and wobbly thighs for years.
Perhaps you've tried every lotion, potion, diet or wonder-
supplement going. And have yet to see results. Or perhaps you've
just been ignoring those podgy, pudgy, orange peely dimples
creeping down your thighs. Maybe you're resigned to it, believing
it's part of a woman's lot.

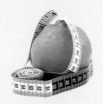

Nearly all women over 20, even supermodels and A list Hollywood
celebs (if those paparazzi shots are anything to go by), are carrying
cellulite somewhere on their body. A dimply bottom, or thighs that
take on an unsightly cottage cheese texture when you cross your
legs, makes you feel blobby, unattractive, overweight, out of shape –
and lacking in confidence. It shouldn't, but it does.

We've written this book in an attempt to provide you with some
lasting solutions. The real culprits include being overweight, having
a sedentary lifestyle and a bad diet. And, yes, lifestyle factors such as
smoking, stress, and frying yourself in the sun all contribute.
Shaping up your bum then, involves losing excess weight, taking

more exercise, overhauling your eating habits – more green stuff, less fatty, salty and sugary stuff, and generally cleaning up your lifestyle. We've also got ideas on lotions, potions and salon treatments that can help and cunning tricks for disguising less than perfect butts.

The bad news is we haven't found a miracle cure to iron out the dimples (and erase the years) instantly. But we have uncovered some clever, inexpensive and simple changes that can knock your bottom into better shape in a matter of weeks. Combine these with some ingenious fashion-camouflage and a few savvy body-confidence tricks and you'll see your bottom and thighs in a whole new light. Who knows, you might even learn to love them...

1. Bottom's up

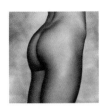

Curves are something to celebrate so try some bottom pampering today.

So before you get stressed, depressed and obsessed about the cellulitey bits, take a moment here to get a perspective, and to celebrate your curves.

■ Savour the good things about your bum and thighs – the excitement of slipping into new silky pants, that satisfying pain/exhilaration when you cycle up a hill or the sensation of rubbing lovely cream into your legs.?

■ Every day, promise yourself you'll do something that makes you feel good about your body – have a manicure, treat yourself a day spa, go for a swim.

■ Make a mental list of your best bits – glossy hair, petite feet, long, beautifully shaped fingernails, firm boobs – and stop focusing on your short-comings.

■ Start taking some exercise. It can boost your mood, improve your complexion, help you focus and give you confidence in your body.

Here's an idea for you...

Toning up you behind doesn't have to
be a full-time occupation. Try this tiny
bum-firming move you can do
anywhere. Raise one foot off the floor
and kick it back behind you in tiny
pulse-moves. Aim for 15 repetitions two
or three times a day.

Defining idea

*'The average girl would rather have
beauty than brains because she knows
the average man can see much better
than he can think.'*
ANON

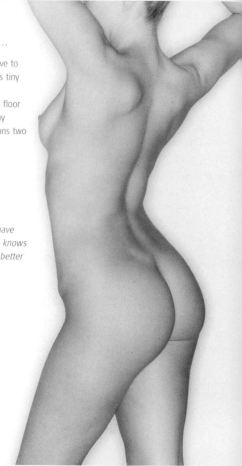

2. Reach your ideal weight

Drop some pounds and you'll shift some cellulite.

Try these five golden rules today to kick start your weight loss:

- Eat breakfast – as long as it's not a fatty fry up. Experts have found that dieters who eat a high fibre breakfast lose more weight than dieters who skip breakfast.
- Make sure you get your five portions of fruit and veg a day. Make them a priority before you eat anything else – you'll feel fuller already and will get more nutrients into your diet.
- Never say never to treats. Depriving yourself of your favourite foods often makes you want to rebel – and you can end up bingeing. Instead, just have a tiny amount and use a teaspoon instead of a dessert spoon. Learn to savour instead of scoff.
- Eat snacks. Healthy snacks – fruit, pitta breads and hummous, nuts and yoghurt help keep your blood sugar levels steady – you won't get hungry, so you're less likely to reach for cakes and chocolate. Aim to eat a low fat snack every two hours.

Here's an idea for you...

Want quick results? Try brushing shimmery bronzer on the backs of legs or thighs or smother thighs with a light-reflecting cream or lotion. They catch the light, making legs look smoother and draw attention away from the cellulitey bits.

■ Watch your portions: some people swear they eat healthily yet never lose weight. Huge portions may be the problem. You should be aiming for no more than a fistful of carbs and protein at one meal. But fill up with plenty of veggies.

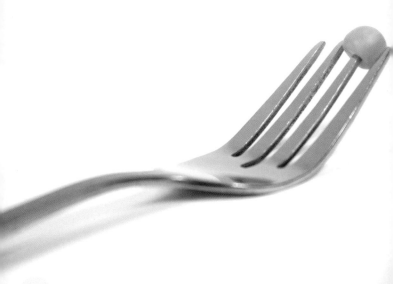

3. Shock treatment

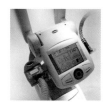

Some women swear by Ionithermie.

Ionithermie is a toning, firming body treatment using electrical charges, which are said to give the muscle a kind of friction-based 'workout', and thereby help firm up your buttocks/thighs too. Some say it's the ideal treatment for those people who have successfully shed the pounds yet still need help to tone and firm. Devotees say it helps with inch loss, and leaves your skin as smooth and silky as the proverbial baby's bottom.

Once you've undressed, the therapist may take measurements from your hips, thighs and bottom before she starts. After your skin is exfoliated you'll be treated to a pressure point massage so you're relaxed before the hard work on your bum really starts. Then your cellulitey bits are covered with a thermal clay and essential oils between layers of gauze. It's cooling and smells delicious. Pads which emit rhythmic electrical pulses are then placed on your skin. When the

Here's an idea for you...

Do some kind of exercise every day. It's good for your skin, your circulation, and burns fat; studies have shown people who raise their heartbeat during exercise more three times a week have improved skin elasticity. Start small, take the stairs instead of the lift, park your car further from the shops, get off the bus a stop earlier.

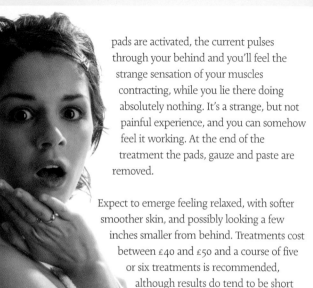

pads are activated, the current pulses through your behind and you'll feel the strange sensation of your muscles contracting, while you lie there doing absolutely nothing. It's a strange, but not painful experience, and you can somehow feel it working. At the end of the treatment the pads, gauze and paste are removed.

Expect to emerge feeling relaxed, with softer smoother skin, and possibly looking a few inches smaller from behind. Treatments cost between £40 and £50 and a course of five or six treatments is recommended, although results do tend to be short term.

Defining idea

'The most wonderful thing about miracles is that they sometimes happen.'
G K CHESTERTON, novelist and essayist

4. Give it the brush-off

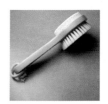

Daily skin brushing can help soften and smooth out orange-peel thighs in days.

Regular body brushing can dramatically enhance the texture of your skin and help the dimples become less noticeable. You can do it every day in the comfort and privacy of your own home, it takes no more than three to five minutes of your time, costs nothing – well, about £5 for a decent brush – and you can usually see results within days.

Body brushing can help minimise cellulite in two ways. Firstly it helps remove surface dead cells, which makes the skin on your rear end look smoother and more even textured. Secondly it stimulates circulation and boosts lymphatic drainage – both of these systems are believed to be involved in cellulite.

How to body-brush

Start at your feet and brush your soles, toes and ankles and top of each foot gently but firmly with long sweeping movements. Brush

Here's an idea for you...

Get the circulation in your bottom and thighs going, and smooth the skin at the same time, with a home-made scrub. Mix 2 tablespoons of finely ground oatmeal together with one tablespoon of almond oil. Rub into the skin, then rinse off in the shower.

the front and back of your lower legs, working towards your knees. Then rest your foot against the bath or a chair and brush from your knees to your upper legs and thighs, waist and buttocks using long smooth strokes. Repeat on both legs. Many women get cellulite on their upper arms, so don't neglect your upper body. Start at your wrist and brush your inner arm in upward strokes towards your elbow. Then brush the palm of your hand, then the outer side of your hand, and move up towards the back of your arm. Repeat on the other arm. Follow with gentle circular movements over your stomach and chest. Once you're done shower or jump in the bath to remove the dead surface cells.

5. Stairway to heaven

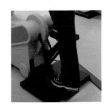

If you want buns of steel try working out on a stepper.

While steppers differ slightly from each other in design and the way they provide resistance, the bottom (sorry) line is that they present you with resistance which you overcome by pressing down or stepping up with alternate legs. To do that your body has to recruit a number of muscles, most notably the gluteus maximus, medius and minimus, known collectively to gym bunnies as the glutes, and to everyone else as your bum. Because of this the stepper is a great means of toning the buttocks – men don't seem to find this important so it's the one piece of equipment we can usually get to use at the gym without too much trouble.

Stairs are hard work because we are supporting our own bodyweight and lifting it up, making each step a mini-lunge or

Here's an idea for you...

As our muscles adapt to an exercise and get better at it they become more efficient and use fewer calories. So keep yourself on your toes by chopping and changing. Most steppers have a random setting which increases or lowers the resistance. Set the machine to 'random' and then cover up the display with a towel so you don't see the changes coming.

Defining idea

'The journey of a thousand miles starts with a single step.'
MAO TSE TUNG, the Great Leader

squat. Up the resistance of the stepper so you have to launch yourself a little harder and you now have a tough workout for the quads at the front of your thighs and the calves at the back of your legs. Upping the resistance also takes the stepper into serious cardio workout territory – which shouldn't come as a surprise to those of us who get out of breath going upstairs – so you can build stamina whilst toning.

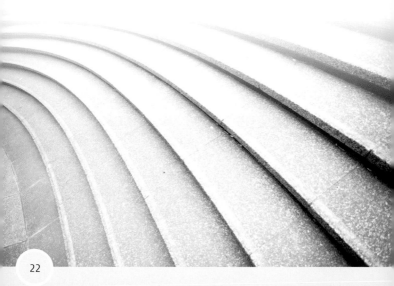

6. Keep on running

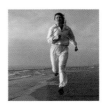

Jogging or even walking is one of the best forms of cellulite-busting exercise.

You don't have to be sporty to fall in love with running. Just take it slowly and keep your goals realistic. Running aids weight loss, is fantastic at toning legs, boosts circulation and helps burn fat and build muscle, so cellulite doesn't stand a chance.

Invest in great workout kit, a diary or notebook and water bottle. You're aiming to do about four workouts a week – but you'll be starting really gently. Always start with five minutes of brisk walking and some stretches to warm up and prepare your body.

Begin by walking regularly, for a couple of weeks or so if you haven't exercised for some time, then start to add short bouts of running to your workout. You're aiming to warm up for five minutes by walking, then run for say 30–60 seconds, then walk for three

Here's an idea for you...

Bin the biscuit tin, and instead snack on a big bowl of grapes; grapes are rich in anthocyanins, which can aid collagen building.

Defining idea

'The only reason I would take up jogging is so that I could hear heavy breathing again.'
ERMA BOMBECK, humorist

minutes, and alternate the pattern. If you start feeling breathless, switch back to walking again. Over a few weeks of workouts, gradually increase your running time and decrease your walking time.

- Keep a progress diary, taking note of your weight and measurements before you begin your new running plan, how you feel after each session – and celebrating each tiny victory.
- Set a goal by signing up for a race, giving yourself at least eight weeks to prepare for it.
- Find a running mate – if you work out with a friend you're more likely to stick to it.
- Get outdoors – studies show that the

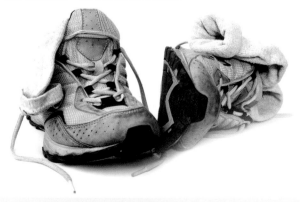

7. Can you feel the force?

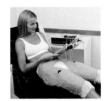

Find out about the massage therapy that can minimise lumps and bumps and reduce thighs by inches.

Endermologie is a special form of deep tissue massage which uses a machine to stretch, stimulate, deep massage and smooth the contours of body fat, thereby reducing the circumference of the thighs or other areas of the body. The machine-based treatment is designed to get to work on the fat pockets that lie beneath the surface skin and which cause you all those problems. As the machine rolls back and forth across the cellulite-ridden area, it sucks in the skin, which helps loosen and break down some of the fat cells. It also helps boost circulation, and stretch the collagen fibres making them more elastic. Meanwhile, the fat is spread into a smooth layer, reducing the lumpy, bumpy appearance.

Here's an idea for you...

If you're unlucky enough to have a man who asks you what you are going to do about your orange peel thighs, ditch him. Save yourself for someone who'll make you feel god about yourself.

25

Defining idea

'A beautiful woman and a wooden boat are very expensive in maintenance.'
Dutch Proverb

Once you've undressed, the therapist helps you don a sort of elasticated body stocking. Then, using a sort of hand held machine, almost like a dustbuster-cum-iron, she massages the skin. Surprisingly, given that the machine is giving your wobbly bits a thorough pummelling, endermologie is actually pleasant. The pain comes when it's time to pay! A 35 minute session will set you back about £70.

In trials, testers found it reduced the circumference of their thighs and hips. One study showed that after having seven treatments, patients lost about 1.34cms from their thighs – and these results were effective even if the patients hadn't actually lost any weight.

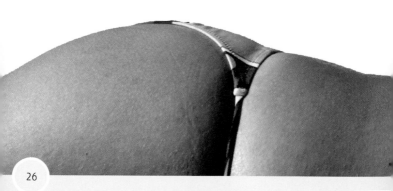

8. Cream's crackers

Moisturising's the No 1 beauty rule, and experts say keeping skin hydrated can help banish those dimples.

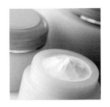

When you slather on moisturiser, it helps plump out your skin. The effects may be temporary but adding moisture can smooth out those dimples and orange peel bits to a degree. When your skin lacks moisture, it looks thinner, so those little pockets of fatty cells beneath the skin (which are the cellulite) are more noticeable. If you re-hydrate your skin, you reduce the appearance of cellulite. Aim to moisturise day and night – after a shower in the morning and before bed. Expensive, delicious smelling unguents make it a more pleasurable task, but any good moisturiser or body oil will do the trick.

There are many specialist cellulite creams out there. These days many products are impressively endorsed by various scientific studies, many of

Here's an idea for you...

Avocadoes are good for your skin. They make a delicious snack or a sandwich/salad ingredient. You can even make a moisturising beauty mask with them. Simply mush up two or three avocados into a soft paste and smother over your bottom – massaging it in using circular movements with the avocado stone. Then just wash it off with warm water.

Defining idea

'I love to put on lotion. Sometimes I'll watch TV and go into a lotion trance for an hour. I try to find brands that don't taste bad in case anyone wants to taste me.'
ANGELINA JOLIE

which claim that testers lost inches and pounds after using the said unguent for a period of time. But cellulite creams alone, however impressive, aren't likely to transform fleshy saggy buttocks into a nectarine-firm bottom.

However they may help more than ordinary moisturisers. Many cellulite creams also contain temporary toning ingredients, which help improve skin texture. Effects can be pretty immediate but are temporary – good for a hot date, beach day, black dress occasion, that sort of thing.

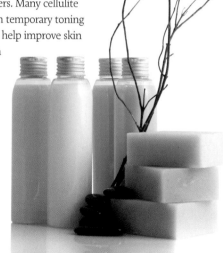

9. Stepping up a gear

Step is a full-on cardio workout to music that firms the thighs, shapes the bum and hones the hamstrings.

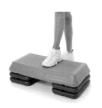

A lot of women decide on the spot that they are either too uncoordinated or too unfit to take part in the choreographed stampede of a step class. But if you want to shape up your bum step is a great class to try out.

Steps of any kind are a surprisingly hard workout – so make sure you start with a beginners' class: step is hard enough work without the stress of playing catch-up. You'll probably warm up with some nice simple side-to-side movements, a bit of stretching as you sway, and some step up/downs. Then the pace will gradually pick up with new moves being added such as stepping

Here's an idea for you...

As you get used to step it gets easier, reducing the benefits of the workout. Progress to the next level offered by your gym as soon as you find that you know what move comes next, you're not as breathless or sweaty as you used to be, or you just fancy something new. If the new class is too much for you, then simply skip some of the moves to keep up – you'll get it in the end.

Defining idea

'To get fit, be fit, and stay fit, one had to be consistent, yet consistently change.'
GIN MILLER, STEP PRIESTESS

sideways on the step, stepping down on the other side, stepping over the step with a twirl to face the other way. The whole thing is done to a strong beat and you may be surprised by how much you sweat. Step is one of those things where it gets easier the better you get at it. As a newbie you are putting in more effort, and getting more of a workout, than the more slick-looking steppers around you. Keep up the good work and marvel as your bottom becomes more pert.

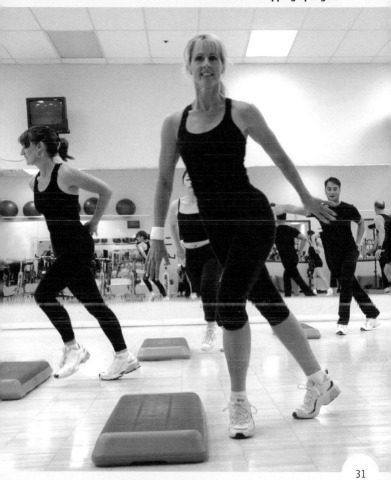

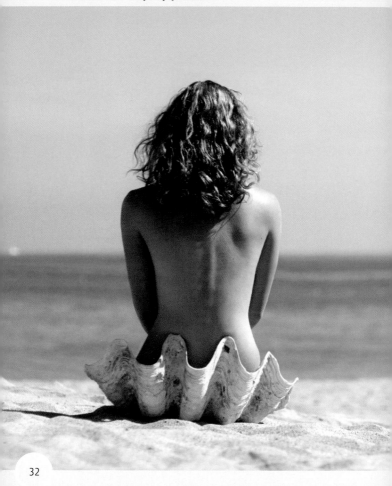

10. Sea nymphs

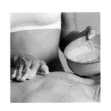

Get the low-down on seaweed and algae body wraps.

Marine products are thought to help with cellulite by boosting circulation and encouraging fluid loss from the skin; so if you think your own cellulite is caused by water retention, it's worth investing in some of the green stuff.

Body wraps have long been used as a cellulite treatment. The process goes something like this; you go to a salon and undress, then a therapist applies some kind of blue, green or browny marine-based mud, then wraps your waist and bottom up in foil, or cling film or some kind of gauze. Thus trussed, you're left gazing at the ceiling or floor, for about an hour, after which you're cleaned, moisturised and sent out into the world, inches smaller and with smoother, firmer skin.

Here's an idea for you...

Swimming's a great all over exercise that can burn fat and calories, boost your skin tone and firm your wobbly bits at the same time. If you don't fancy swimming next time you're at the beach, walking through waist high water is also great for toning the muscles in your legs.

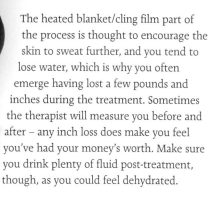

The heated blanket/cling film part of the process is thought to encourage the skin to sweat further, and you tend to lose water, which is why you often emerge having lost a few pounds and inches during the treatment. Sometimes the therapist will measure you before and after – any inch loss does make you feel you've had your money's worth. Make sure you drink plenty of fluid post-treatment, though, as you could feel dehydrated.

It's not a miracle solution, as the pounds will return as you drink to replenish the lost fluids. But if you're beach-bound, look upon it as a temporary cellulite-minimiser or tummy flattener. Plus it's actually fairly pleasant – deeply relaxing, and wonderfully pampering. And, appearance aside, the products usually smell delectable.

Defining idea

'Eternity begins and ends with the ocean's tides.'
ANON

11. I want muscles

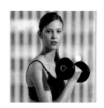

Muscle-building exercise can boost your metabolic rate and help you burn more body fat, which means less cellulite.

Lean muscle fills out your skin, so saggy cellulite tissue could be transformed into neat, toned, smoother, taut buttocks in a matter of weeks. When you work on building and firming your muscles and reducing body fat, it helps effectively lift the skin, which can help prevent that puckering which takes place when the fibres pull downwards. In fact, one study found that 70% of women said their cellulite improved in just 6 weeks by doing weight training on their legs.

The trouble with muscle is that when we reach our late 30s, we start losing it whilst gaining fat, even if our diet stays the same. So you may find your cellulite has become more noticeable over the years.

Working with weight machines, dumbbells, barbells, body bars, body bands, wrist or ankle weights constitutes an effective resistance workout, so head for your local gym and ask a trainer to devise a workout for you.

Here's an idea for you...

Is water retention making your wobbly bits puffy? Try eating lots of natural diuretics such as celery, onion, parsley, aubergines, garlic and peppermint.

The aim is to build in three sessions of resistance work a week. Outside the gym, walking or cycling with ankle weights, doing squats and lunges or taking part in spinning or step classes will all help build muscle.

Stick to low fat foods, with plenty of fresh fruit and veg. Lean protein is important for muscles, as it helps repair the muscle fibres you may have damaged. So eat plenty of chicken, fish, dairy –tofu, lentils, nuts. Spread your protein evenly over 5 or 6 meals a day to maximise absorption and minimise fat gain. If you're working out three times a week you need about 5–7g of carbs per kg of body weight daily. Remember to include calcium-rich foods such as dairy, beans and green leafy vegetables to help support your bones.

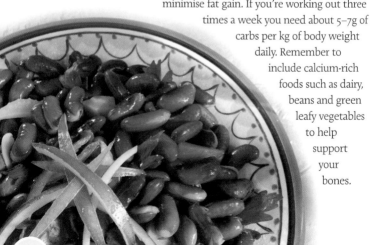

12. Goodbye Mr Chips

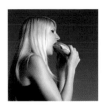

Cut back on fat and you'll reap rewards on your bum and thighs.

You don't have to suffer on a fat-free regime to lose weight. There are plenty of painless ways to cut back. Try sticking to a moderate fat restriction eating plan, where it accounts for 30–35% of your total calorie intake. You're much more likely to keep the weight off than with more severe restrictions because it's more palatable and therefore easier to stick with. Try the following:

- Ban margarine, butter or cheese in your sandwiches;
- Reduce red meat consumption by using beans, fish or lean white meat instead;
- Keep away from foods preserved in oil; stick to brine or freshwater instead;
- Stop frying food; instead barbecue/griddle or grill your fish or meat;
- Never add cream to pasta sauces or soups;

Here's an idea for you...

Can't say no to afternoon tea? Try munching warmed fruit loaf with your cuppa instead of butter laden crumpets; fruit loaf is rich in fibre and iron and is gooey and moist so you won't need oodles of butter.

Defining idea

'No diet will remove all the fat from your body because the brain is entirely fat. Without a brain, you might look good, but all you could do is run for public office.'
GEORGE BERNARD SHAW

■ Minimise cooking fat by using spray olive oils.

Don't forget your body needs one to two daily servings of essential fatty acids and monounsaturated fats each day for energy, eye function, brain-power and for healthy skin and hair. Fats are also needed to absorb fat-soluble vitamins A, D, E and K which are important for vision, strong bones, and to help fight disease. Good sources include avocado, olive or rapeseed oils, sunflower or pumpkin seeds, walnuts and oily fish such as sardines or mackerel.

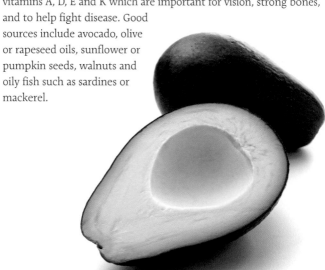

13. Weighty help

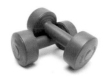

**Here's how hand-held weights can work
your thighs, hamstrings, calves and
buttocks.**

Squats

Start with two dumbbells, one in each hand, at your sides, your feet
shoulder-width apart, knees very slightly bent. With your shoulders
pulled back, bend your knees and ease your body down as if you were
slipping into a comfy chair. Don't go so far down that either your knees
move further forward than your toes, or your bum is so low that your
thighs dip down instead of being parallel to the floor. Go too low and
you risk overextending and straining your muscles. Smoothly raise
yourself back up to the start position. Keep the whole movement
smooth and controlled – don't bounce.

Lunges

Start as with the squat, but this time take a long step forward so your
front foot is now about a yard from your back one. Keeping your torso
upright, lower your body by bending your legs. Your front knee

shouldn't go past your toes. Even though you may feel a burning sensation down the length of your back leg it's the muscles of the front thigh that should be doing the work as you now lift your body back up by straightening the front leg. For a bit of variety try to switch from forward lunges to backward lunges, where you step backwards with one leg before lunging.

Here's an idea for you...

To hit your hip flexors try a sideways lunge. Start in the usual position but with lighter than usual weights (at least until you're used to the exercise) then take a very big step sideways as far as you can reach. Lower yourself by bending the leg that stepped out, keeping your knee moving in the same line as the foot. Smoothly straighten your knee to bring you back, and then step back to the start position.

14. Beans means lines

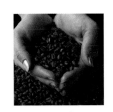

If you're a coffee fiend, here's why it's time to switch to decaf.

Caffeine's thought to contribute to cellulite – for several reasons. It can contribute to weight gain by raising the levels of the stress hormone cortisol and insulin in your body, which is thought to accelerate ageing and encourage the body to store fat. When our blood sugar levels are raised and our insulin levels are disrupted, we're more likely to be tempted by sugary treats – that espresso may lead to a choccy croissant or two.

Caffeine is also bad for your skin because it impedes your blood circulation. Skin requires a regular blood circulation to say looking young and healthy. Too much caffeine will make skin dry and dehydrated making cellulite worse.

Here's an idea for you...

Ditch that coffee and try instead starting your day with a large glass of freshly squeezed orange juice and a bowl of berries. They're packed with vitamin C, which is important for the production of collagen and can strengthen the capillaries, which feed the skin. And better skin can mean smoother thighs.

Defining idea

*'Behind every successful woman is a
substantial amount of coffee'*
STEPHANIE PIRO, artist

Caffeine also contributes to water
retention which, manifested on
your bottom and thighs, makes
your skin bulge out and look
puffier and more dimply.

About 300mg caffeine a day is 'a moderate' intake. One cup of coffee
contains about 100 mg per 190ml, tea 30–60 mg per 190ml cup and
cola around 50 mg per can. Best advice, then, is to cut down as
much as you can – don't drink more than one or two cups a day –
and look instead for healthy alternatives. Chocolate also contains
caffeine – there's more caffeine in a 125g of dark choc than in a cup
of instant coffee...so if you're
serious about getting
rid of cellulite, go
easy on the
chocolate
too.

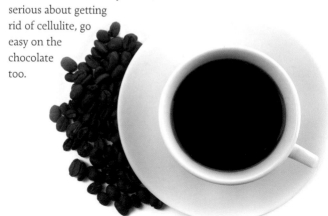

15. Still waters

Water's great for skin, and a few glasses a day may help reduce orange peel thighs.

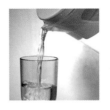

Drinking plenty of water can help beat cellulite on several fronts. It can be a great weight loss tool. Many of us often confuse hunger with thirst, so we end up eating instead of drinking, increasing our calorie intake unnecessarily. Research shows that 75% of all hunger pangs are actually thirst, so if you get the munchies, try a glass of water instead – and save yourself calories.

As a skin enhancer, water works wonders. It helps your body absorb the nutrients from food, which your skin needs to function optimally. When you're dehydrated, your body effectively steals water from your skin to deliver to the more important organs, so skin is the first thing to suffer if you're not drinking enough.

Here's an idea for you...

Make sure you're well hydrated at all times. Carry a bottle around with you and sip regularly. Match every caffeine beverage or alcoholic drink with a glass of water. When you're exercising drink about 2 glasses (400-600ml) 2 to three hours before you start your work out.

Drinking plenty of water can also help beat the water retention that contributes to cellulite. When you're dehydrated, or eat too much sodium, your body's cells hold on to the water they already have, fearing they won't get much more. The result is water swelling in your fat cells, contributing to that dimply bottom look. Fresh fruit, veg and wholegrains will help rebalance the sodium and potassium in your body, and eliminate excess fluid in your fat pockets.

A 60kg adult needs 1.5–2 litres (6–8 250ml glasses) of fluids a day – the majority of which should be water. The colour of your urine is the best gauge – you're after a pale watery colour with a tinge of lemon. Yellow urine means you need to drink more.

Defining idea

'Water is the driving force of all nature.'
LEONARDO DA VINCI

16. Top gear

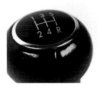

**Calculate your basal metabolic rate (BMR)
and rev up your metabolism.**

BMR = weight in kilos x 2 x 11.

So, if you're 65 kilos, your BMR = 65 x 2 x 11 = 1430

Now work out how many extra calories you expend as a result of the
activity you take:

■ inactive or sedentary – BMR x 20%
■ you walk and take exercise once or twice a week – BMR x 30%
■ you exercise two or three times a week – BMR x 40%
■ you exercise hard more than 3 times a week – BMR x 50%
■ you exercise hard every day – BMR x 70%

So if you're a fairly active 65kg woman – 1430 x 30% = 429

Add these two together to find out how many calories you need a
day: 1430 + 429 = 1859. Eat more than this without increasing your
activity levels and you'll gain weight.

To boost your metabolic rate:

■ Exercise. When you increase the amount of lean tissue in your body,
  you use up more calories even when you're just sitting there since
  muscle uses more calories than fat.

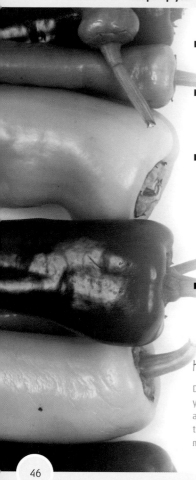

- Eat protein. The body uses more calories metabolising protein than other foodstuffs.
- Add some chillies to your dishes – apparently they can raise your metabolic rate by about 50% for up to two or three hours after a meal.
- Have a pre- and post-exercise nibble. A study found that people who performed gentle resistance exercise within two hours of eating a light carb-based meal boosted their metabolic rate, and burned the food off quicker than those who didn't exercise afterwards.
- Drink green tea. Studies show that drinking two cups daily could help you burn about 70 calories more each day.

Here's an idea for you...

Drinking two litres of still water a day can help your body burn off an extra 150 calories according to one study. It's thought to stimulate the sympathetic nervous system and increase the metabolic rate.

17. In a spin

If you like the idea of long lean legs and taut buttocks, then it's time to brave the Spinning studio.

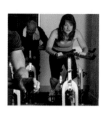

Spinning is the closest you can get to partying in the saddle and the fierce calorie burn (up to double normal cycling on your own) plus the toning of hamstrings, calves, hips and abs adds up to quite a workout.

Classes start with some nice easy warm-up exercises to get you used to the feel of the bike, and to give you an idea of what's in store. There are three basic moves – sprints, climbs and jumps. Sprints are exactly what they sound like – the instructor encourages you to set a level of resistance and then burn away as fast as you can. Climbs mean a high level of resistance and standing on the pedals to keep it moving. Jumps mean short, sharp spells out of the saddle.

The instructor will encourage you to turn the resistance up and down depending on the 'road'

Here's an idea for you...

Spinning is pretty intensive so it pays to show up prepared. Of all the classes you've ever done this is the one where you'll suffer if you don't have a water bottle to hand. Spin bikes have a water holder on the handlebars or frame so just stop every now and again and glug.

Defining idea

*'When I see an adult on a
bicycle, I do not despair of the
future of the human race.'*
H.G. WELLS

ahead. Your gym will provide
stomping music, perhaps darken
the room, and maybe even put on a
light show. The emphasis is on an
all-singing all-dancing total
absorption into the moment and
the result is great fun. If you're
worried that the pace is likely to
be too hectic for you, don't be.
It's up to you how much you
increase the resistance – your
instructor's legs may spin like a
washing machine but that
doesn't mean you should follow
suit straight away.

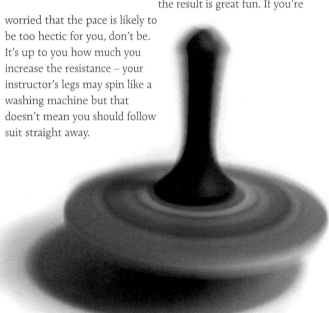

18. Brown girl in the ring

Cellulite looks less obvious on bronzed legs. If you can't beat it...hide it with a fake tan!

A home fake tan tends to last up to four or five days. Salon tans are less hassle and tend to last longer – some claim theirs last as much as a fortnight. Many fake tans take a few days to look beautifully natural, so if you're preparing for a special do, book your treatment a few days prior to the event.

If you don't fancy a salon treatment follow this self tanning guide. Make sure you patch test your skin beforehand to avoid an allergic reaction. Don't be tempted to go too dark; always choose one that matches your natural skin tone.

Here's an idea for you...

Need to lose a few pounds? Start your meal with soup. Studies show that tucking into a bowl of soup before a meal can fill you up, so you're less likely to overeat. Try a high water based soup, broth-style with plenty of veggies.

Defining idea

Start by exfoliating with a body
scrub, loofah or flannel. Apply
exfoliator with circular movements,
paying particular attention to heels,
knees and elbows where the skin is
rougher. Always moisturise after
exfoliating and leave the
moisturiser on for about 15 minutes before you apply your fake tan.
Remove excess moisturiser with a damp flannel before you apply –
especially on bony areas such as knees, elbows and ankles – it'll
prevent any uneven tanning. Apply the fake tan, smothering it on as
you would a moisturiser. Don't forget backs of knees, inner thighs,
backs of your hands. You don't need as much where your skin is
thinner as the colour will stay longer here. Tan usually appears
about three or four hours later – if you find you have streaks, try
exfoliating the area.

Avoid swimming or having a shower for about 12 hours after a
treatment. Moisturise your body well over the next few days; it'll
help prolong your fake tan. And always remember that a fake tan
won't protect you from the sun so you still need sunscreen.

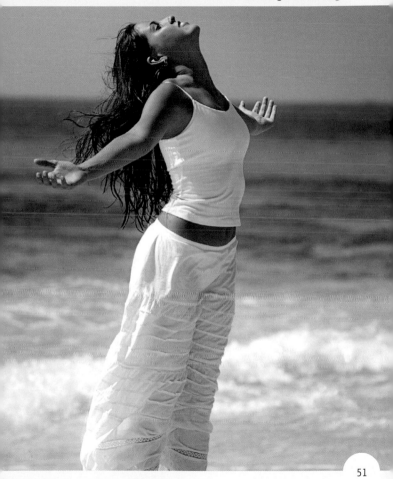

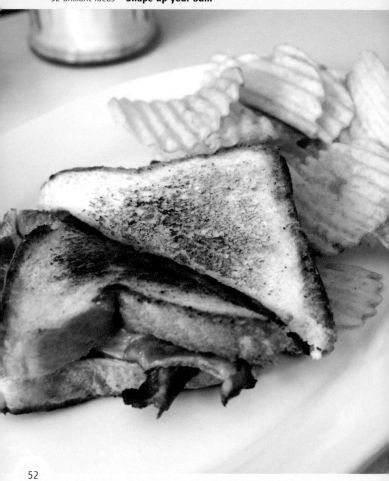

19. There's a rat in the kitchen

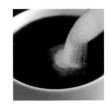

Additives, salt and sugar all conspire to make your bottom crinkly, so start saying no to processed foods.

Salt encourages your body to hold on to water, causing bloating and the dimpling under the skin that we know as cellulite. Watch your salt intake – have no more than 6g of salt or 2.5 of sodium a day. Cut back on processed foods including stock, sauces and soups and cook from scratch instead. Aim to drink plenty of fluids every day (at least eight glasses) and potassium-rich fruit and veg, to help dilute the salt. Use fresh herbs, spices, or lemon to flavour your food instead.

Sugar is high in calories, and when we eat sugary foods, it can cause blood sugar levels to surge, triggering the release of insulin and encouraging fat storage. A high sugar diet has also been linked to premature skin ageing; it has an inflammatory effect on our tissues and can cause the collagen to become hard and less elastic. Too-taut collagen in your skin can contribute to the puckering effect on your bottom and thighs. Rather than banning sweet treats limit them to a once weekly indulgence. Search labels for hidden sugars including

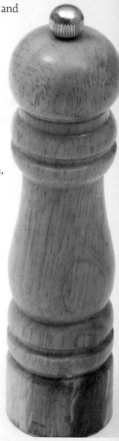

Here's an idea for you...

If you want to minimise the cellulite while posing for holiday snaps, hold yourself in a way that disguises excess curves; stand up and pivot slightly on your feet so your body including your shoulders is at a slight angle. Put your hands on your hips to make your waist look smaller.

glucose syrup and dextrose and aim for foods with less than 2g sugar per 100g. Swap soft drinks for water, smoothies and natural juices and sweeten foods with fresh, stewed or dried fruit.

Some scientists claim that the pesticide residues and additives found in many foods, actually interfere with our metabolism, disrupt our hormone balance and increase our appetite, all of which can make us gain pounds. So choose fresh, organic foods where possible. Keep your fat intake, especially animal fats, down (pesticides accumulate in fats). Eat plenty of soluble fibre found in pulses, grains, fruit and veg to soak up chemicals from other foods. Cut back on savoury snacks, desserts, sweets and snack bars – they're often full of colours, preservatives or additives.

20. Be a mistress of disguise

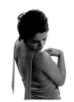

Some clothes actually draw attention to cellulite. Learn what to wear to make the most of your assets.

The first rule is to wear the right size clothes for your body. In fact if you're trying to hide a generous bottom and saddlebag thighs, you could even wear a size bigger than you actually are; trousers will hang more flatteringly, making you look neater and trimmer.

A spongy bottom can be camouflaged with a few wardrobe classics. Stick to side-fastening trousers instead of front-fastening ones. Wear long jackets instead of cropped ones; they'll cover your behind. And don't be tempted by drainpipe trousers; stick to wide legs that make your tush altogether more petite. Hipsters are a big-bottomed girl's best friend as they create the illusion of having smaller hips. But avoid an expanse of flesh 'overhang' as it can ruin the effect – team them with a floaty top. Experiment with a boot leg cut – it's even more flattering as it makes your legs look longer and slimmer.

Defining idea...

'If love is blind, why is lingerie so popular?'
Anon

Tailored clothes tend to look better on generously proportioned behinds so splash out on some quality classics – you'll notice the difference instantly. Tailored flares, floaty palazzo pants and A-line skirts are great for disguising cellulitey bottoms and thighs and saddlebags.

In general
- stick to small patterns rather than unflattering big ones
- avoid panty lines at all costs
- never wear leggings or spray on lycra – boy, can it show up the bulges
- stick to floaty fabrics such as chiffon or tailored lines in natural fibres such as linen or cotton
- seek out textured fabrics, which can help to 'break up' flesh. Try linen, wool or even crinkled man made fabrics.

Here's an idea for you...

Draw the eye away from your rear end by dressing up your top half – gorgeous billowy tops in bold colours can take unwanted attention away from your thighs.

21. Squatters' rights

Squats tone up your thighs, hips, calves and buttocks.

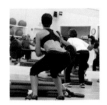

Squats train your body in balance, they strengthen the stabilisers and tone the thighs and buttocks. They can increase your flexibility and range of movement and even protect your back from the wear and tear of daily life. So much from so little.

Start off with your feet shoulder-width apart and your legs very lightly bent at the knee. Breathe in and pull your shoulders back a little so that your spine assumes its natural curve in your lower back. You may find it more comfortable to open the stance slightly by pointing your toes outwards. Just remember that your knees must move in the same axis as your feet, so toes outwards means your knees move outwards too – otherwise you'll risk strain.

With your arms out straight in front of you like a sleepwalker, bend your knees and ease yourself down as if sitting into an armchair. The lift is done by straightening those knees and driving down through the legs and heels. Keep the whole sole of your foot firmly planted

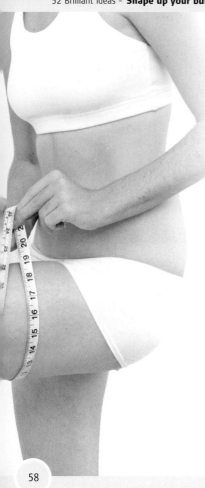

on the floor. Do three sets of twelve reps. Once you're comfortable doing squats without weight, try a broomstick held across the back of your shoulders. Watch yourself in the mirror as you squat to ensure your head and neck are straight up and the natural curve of your spine isn't exaggerated as you work.

Here's an idea for you...

If your heels rise off the floor as you lower into the squat pause at the bottom of the squat and place your heels firmly on the floor before driving upwards. In addition try calf stretches. Stand on a step with both feet together, balls of the feet on the edge of the step, heels out in space. Now pivoting with the middle of your sole on the edge of the step, lower one heel at a time and feel the stretch.

22. Come to bed thighs

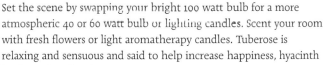

Nothing cools a woman's ardour more than the thought of a man coming face to face with her cellulitey body. So make the bedroom work for you.

Set the scene by swapping your bright 100 watt bulb for a more atmospheric 40 or 60 watt bulb or lighting candles. Scent your room with fresh flowers or light aromatherapy candles. Tuberose is relaxing and sensuous and said to help increase happiness, hyacinth has been found to increase sensuality and fragrances such as jasmine, ylang ylang, patchouli, sandalwood, rose, cardamom, cedarwood, cinnamon and clary sage are known for their aphrodisiac qualities. Dress the bed with fantastic crisp, cotton sheets, throws, fur blankets and plump cushions (which you can strategically place over yourself). Have mellow music ready.

Here's an idea for you...

Hot day? Hot date? If you want to reveal some flesh without displaying your cellulitey arms or legs, show off your back instead. Try a backless dress or long-sleeved top with a plunging back. Keep your back looking toned (with exercise) and smooth; exfoliate regularly with a long-handled loofah, and soak in moisturising bath oils.

Defining idea...

'My wife was afraid of the dark ... then she saw me naked and now she's afraid of the light.'
RODNEY DANGERFIELD, comedian

Look less lumpy instantly by improving your posture; imagine a string pulling you up from the centre of your head. Your stomach should be pressed flat and your shoulders relaxed down into your back. If there's time, try a twenty minute workout before your date; by boosting your circulation you'll improve skin tone and look more radiant. Set aside five or ten minutes to exfoliate your skin to remove surface dead skin cells, then moisturise; it'll help 'plump' up the skin. Make use of bronzer and moisturising creams with light reflecting particles; these can make legs look more even textured and glowing.

In terms of bedroom attire don't go too skimpy. Always buy knickers and bras in the correct size so you're not spilling over the top. Satin is great as it skims over your bumps. Distract from the dimply bottom by drawing the eye to other bits; for example you could wear a beautiful necklace or choker.

23. The big chill

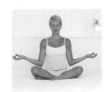

The stress hormone cortisol can make cellulite worse. Time for some simple stress–reduction strategies.

Stress can contribute to cellulite on several levels. Firstly, long-term stress can make you fat because it often increases the appetite for carbohydrate rich 'comfort' foods. The hormone cortisol, which is released when you are stressed, can increase fat storage in the abdominal area (where many of us get cellulite). Stress can also compromise your overall nutrition because it makes the food pass more quickly through the digestive system, which means less of it is actually absorbed. Finally stress causes hormonal changes in your body, affecting the function of cells in your vital organs which is reflected in the appearance of your skin. So try some of these tips to de-stress:

- Make sure you relax five or ten minutes before meals to prepare your digestive system; food will be absorbed and metabolised more efficiently if you're calmer.

Here's an idea for you...

Have a laugh. Studies show people who laugh have significantly lower levels of adrenalin. Watch some funny videos or get your friends over regularly for a fun evening.

Defining idea...

'Stress: the confusion created when one's mind overrides the body's basic desire to choke the living daylights out of some jerk who desperately deserves it'
ANONYMOUS

- Don't let chores get on top of you. Write achievable, realistic to-do list – for daily/weekly/monthly chores.
- Keep your surroundings de-cluttered: every day have a 15 minute tidy up before bedtime – put your clothes out for the morning, make sure the supper dishes are cleaned up and put away.
- Get some exercise: ideally try to manage 30 minutes of moderate exercise at least 5 days of the week.
- Pamper yourself with a haircut, manicure or massage.
- Perfect a mantra: in times of stress or anxiety, take five minutes out for some meditation. Silently repeat a soothing word or phrase, such as 'peace,' while taking slow, deep breaths through your nose.

24. Gold fingers

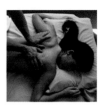

Manual lymphatic drainage (MLD) is described as the best massage treatment there is for cellulite – so lie back and enjoy!

MLD is not the kind of massage that gets knots out of tense muscles or boosts blood flow, but instead uses gentle, rhythmic movements to stimulate the body's lymphatic system making it more efficient at ridding the body of toxins, waste and excess fluid, and improving the circulation of nutrients. Via the lymph system, waste products are carried to the lymph nodes, which are like cleansing stations, located in the neck, armpits, abdomen and groin. The harmful substances are processed in the nodes before entering the bloodstream and being carried on to the liver for detoxification and excretion.

MLD is primarily linked to the reduction of cellulite through the elimination of excess fluid (or water retention). Additionally cellulite may be partly caused by the build up of toxins, so it makes sense that the lymphatic system, which helps remove waste products from the body, could play an important role in reducing it.

Here's an idea for you...

Give yourself a massage. Try massaging your legs and bottom with essential oil of sandalwood; it's a lovely lubricating oil that's very nourishing for dehydrated skin. It's also great for helping you sleep and for relieving anxiety. Add a drop or two to 15-20ml carrier oil such as grapeseed or almond.

During a session the therapist uses gentle rhythmic pumping movements to move the skin in the direction of the lymph flow, so that the lymph moves more freely towards the nodes. Treatment always includes the neck, because lymph nodes are located there, and for cellulite the buttocks, thighs and abdomen will also be targetted. Treatments last about an hour, and usually cost slightly more than other forms of massage because of the highly specialised nature of the training involved.

Defining idea...

'Why do we pay for psychotherapy when massages cost half as much?'
JASON LOVE

Make sure you are treated by a member of the Association of Manual Lymphatic Drainage Practitioners (MLDUK). Find a practitioner at www.mlduk.org.uk.

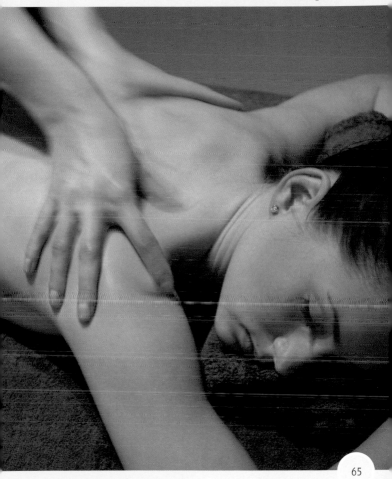

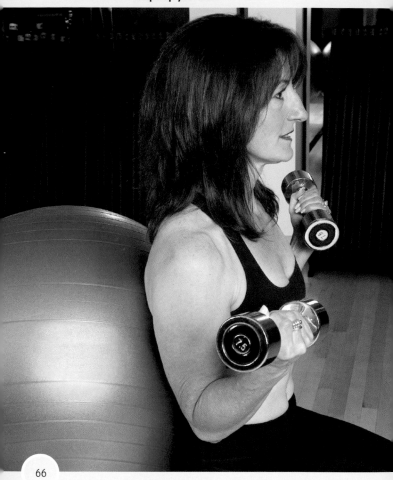

25. Balls to the wall

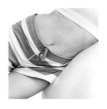

Combining the wall with the Swiss ball can provide a workout for the thighs and bum while keeping the back beautifully supported.

Tuck the Swiss ball behind you between your back and wall so that it pushes naturally into the curve of your spine. Make sure your feet are hip width apart and flat on the floor, with the knees very slightly bent. The feet should be placed a good foot length or more ahead of you so that as you bend your legs the kneecaps do not go further forward than your foot. Slide your shoulder blades back and down, scoop your stomach, and breathing in, bend the knees and feel your back and ball moving down the wall. Don't go down so far that either your knees go further forward than your foot, or your bum drops lower than your knees.

Now exhale and move back up to the start point, feeling the pressure in your thigh muscles. Make sure you resist the temptation to lock the knees at the top of the movement. Make sure you take

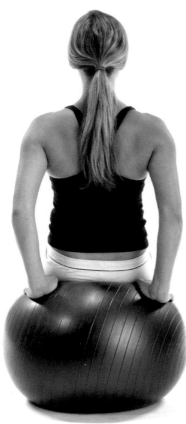

equally long on both the upwards and downwards movement because they are both strength builders but for different muscles. Six repetitions should be enough.

To work your inner thighs, begin as for the normal squat but with the feet placed slightly wider than shoulder-width and the toes pointed very slightly outwards. Don't try to place your legs too wide at first, however, or you'll do yourself a mischief.

Here's an idea for you...

Try squatting with your ankles closer together and the toes pointing apart in what dancers call a small turnout. Make sure you turn out from the hips to avoid injury. Six repetitions should be enough to prepare you for Swan Lake.

26. Cigarettes and alcohol

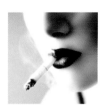

Smoking, drinking, late nights and wild living may be thrilling, but they're utterly bad news for thighs. Here's why.

Some of the great things you're doing to reduce your cellulite will be wiped out the next time you light up. Smoking deprives the skin of nutrients, and free radicals produced by smoking reduce the elasticity of collagen in your skin, creating wrinkles and sagging and allowing fat cells to bulge out between the collagen fibres.

Long-term alcohol abuse can lead to several serious diseases as well as putting women at greater risk of sexual and physical attack. At the very least it can cause weight gain and premature ageing – and make cellulite worse. That's because alcohol can reduce your circulation and cause dehydration, robbing the skin of moisture and vital nutrients. Alcohol can disrupt your sleep, making you too tired for your cellulite-busting workout, and can also dent your self-control so

Defining idea...

'Bad habits are like a comfortable bed, easy to get into, but hard to get out of.'
PROVERB

Here's an idea for you...

Ask 10 of the friends who keep nagging you to give up smoking to put their money where their mouths are. Get them to bet you £10 that you can't go a month without a cigarette. Think of the agony of having to shell out £100 if you fail, and if you win (of course you will!) use the money to treat yourself to some pampering anti-cellulite treatments. And if you've gone a month without lighting up, you know you can crack it for good.

you're more likely to be tempted by junk food. On top of all that, alcohol calories can't be stored by the body, but have to be used as they are consumed – this means that calories excess to requirements from other foods get stored as fat instead.

So that's just one more reason to limit your drinking and give up the smokes.

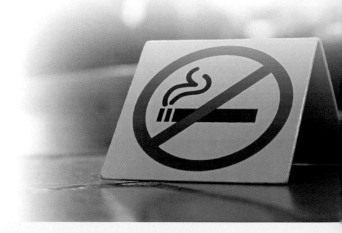

27. Getting a skinful

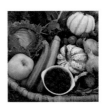

Certain foods contain skin-boosting nutrients that help keep the tissues between the fat cells supple, which can help minimise cellulite. Here's what to put on your plate.

Essential fatty acids help produce collagen, keeping your skin firm and those fat cells in place; great for improving the elasticity and texture of skin. Found in oily and cold water fish (including salmon, tuna and mackerel), olive oil, flaxseed oil, nuts and seeds.

Fruits and veggies are rich in antioxidants that help fight the free radicals that can lead to wrinkles. Choose at least five portions of varied brightly coloured fruits and veg a day. Berries are particularly high in antioxidants and great for skin health.

Lean protein is essential for making collagen and low in fat. Include turkey, chicken, skimmed milk, eggs and soya products such as tofu.

Here's an idea for you...

Keep your tummy feeling fuller for longer by choosing the most filling foods, calorie per calorie. Studies show that potatoes are twice as filling as grain bread, porridge or oatmeal is twice as filling as muesli, oranges are almost twice as filling as bananas and crackers are twice as filling as croissants!

Defining idea...

'Worthless people live only to eat and drink; people of worth eat and drink only to live.'
SOCRATES

Broccoli, cauliflower and cabbage are good for keeping your digestive system working properly and stimulating the liver to remove waste and toxins from the body. When you lighten your toxic load, your skin looks better.

Lecithin is known for its ability to repair skin tissues. It's found in eggs, soya, cauliflower, organ meats, spinach, lettuce and tomatoes.

B Vitamins help your body utilise other cellulite-busting ingredients. Good sources include dark leafy veg, low fat dairy foods, fish, eggs, beans and wholegrains.

Circulation-boosting foods deliver your skin cells a regular supply of life giving nutrients and oxygen; good foods include onions, garlic, nuts, pumpkin seeds and fish.

Vitamin E rich foods promote healing and protect skin by maintaining cells. Found in sweet potatoes, avocadoes, vegetable oils, sunflower seeds, wheat germ, sweetcorn, cashews, almonds and peanuts.

28. With a thong in my heart

The right swimwear can flatter even the most dimply behind. Follow these four rules, and you can still get almost-naked with confidence.

1. Rebalance. If you're bottom heavy, rebalance your silhouette with mix and match. To minimise a curvaceous bum, try a dark solid colour on the bottom and put the colour and pattern on top. Balance out a flat chest with a bandeau style bikini.

2. Disguise. Fake tan is a must. Look for suntan cream with fake tan base and pack on afterwards with a tan prolonger. The browner those cheeks look, the smoother they'll appear. Watch the pattern on your swim-wear. Large motifs tend to make you look fleshier than you are, so make sure any motif is smaller than your fist. String ties are actually more flattering than too tight cuts that make hips and thighs bulge over the top. Flippy skirt bottoms are great for camouflaging thick cellulitey thighs.

Here's an idea for you...

Capitalise on exotic fresh fruits when at your holiday buffet. Fill your plate with yummy papaya and pineapple; they contain a compound called bromelain, which can help beat bloating.

3. Enhance. Put your other assets on display. Give yourself a great pre bikini shape up by applying some bust firming creams. The results tend to be temporary but they can help firm up a sagging décolletage and boost elasticity. Draw more attention to your boobs with padded bras, frilly bits, bright colours, horizontal stripes, or try underwired shapes with bows or flowers for extra oomph.

4. Distract. Accessories are a great way to distract the eye from the bits you don't want to display. Invest in a flowing kaftan, stylish beach bag, and dainty jewellery. A pair of wedge-soled sandals or espadrilles gives you extra inches to make you feel leggy and willowy – and instantly more attractive. Paint your toe-nails beautifully, blow dry your hair or pin up tendrils for water-baby glamour.

Defining idea...

'An optimist is a girl who mistakes a bulge for a curve.'
RING LARDNER, writer

29. The power of lovely lingerie

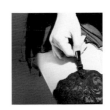

Choose underwear that makes the most of your bum and you feel great.

There are days when those cotton no-frills knickers work well. But for a confidence boost there's something empowering about something more luxurious

Sex appeal has a lot to do with confidence and there is nothing like good underwear to enhance your body shape and make you feel more attractive. A sexy g-string can work wonders for your buttocks. Some people find them incredibly uncomfortable but once you get used to them you will hardly ever wear ordinary knickers again. To make sure you don't suffer from the dreaded VPL under trousers always make sure you have a few g-strings. If you really don't get on with strings try french knickers or boxer shorts for girls – no VPL and damn sexy!

Defining idea...

'A lady is one who never shows her underwear unintentionally.'
LILLIAN DAY, American author

Here's an idea for you...

Fancy underwear is all very well, but a pain to hand wash. So take it into the shower with you and wash it there, which is much easier. It also means you don't end up with that awful grey shade of white as your smalls get washed on a 60 degree cycle with all the wrong colours. Treat it well, and it will last much longer.

If you're wearing the right underwear, you feel like you can take on the world. It makes you feel so much more confident. You walk into a business meeting or social gathering and although the others can't see what you've got on underneath your outfit, you know, and it gives you a sense of superiority. For more intimate encounters the great thing about sexy underwear is that it enhances your sex drive as well as your partner's. You're hardly going to sit around feeling unattractive and worrying about wobbles in a luxurious creation of lace and satin.

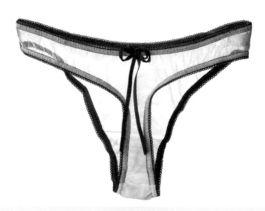

30. Food of the gods (and goddesses)

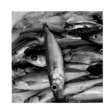

Protein helps build muscles, boosts your metabolism and fills you up. Here's why cellulite hates it.

1. It can aid weight loss by helping to keep your blood sugar levels steady, meaning you stay feeling fuller for longer. It also helps prevent sugar cravings, so you'll be less likely to be tempted by sweet treats.

2. It contains important amino acids which help produce fresh collagen, so it's good for your skin – whether it's on your face or your behind. Keeping your skin in great condition means the cellulite is less noticeable.

3. It helps build muscle. By increasing your muscle mass, you'll boost your metabolic rate, and your body will become more efficient at burning off calories.

Here's an idea for you...

Want a simple, low calone appetite suppressant? Try a snack of houmous and an oatcake or crispbread. It's an instant energy booster, and a great way to rebalance your blood sugar levels and fill you up till supper time.

4. It contains a substance called albumin, which helps absorb excess fluid in your tissues. Water retention around the thighs and bottom is another oft-quoted cause of cellulite.

About 15–20% of your diet should come from proteins and you should aim to eat three portions a day. Women need about 45g of protein each day.

155g portion of lean rump steak = 44g protein
85g portion lean roast chicken = 26g protein
130g grilled cod steak = 27g protein
boiled egg = 8g protein
40g cheddar cheese = 10g protein
200g tin baked beans = 10g protein
30g peanuts = 7g protein

Proteins with benefits:
Animal proteins such as meat, poultry, fish and dairy produce contain all the eight essential amino acids your body needs. Plant foods such as nuts, pulses and grains are great source of low fat protein but because none of them contains all eight essential amino acids vegetarians need to eat a variety of these foods daily to ensure they get a full compliment of amino acids.

31. Scents of a woman

Natural remedies, essential oils and aromatherapy treatments can help reduce cellulite.

Certain essential oils have therapeutic properties which can help regulate your hormones (oestrogen is thought to be a contributing factor both to cellulite and to being overweight), others are great for the skin, and some have effective diuretic qualities so they can help beat water retention, which many of us blame for our bulgy thighs.*

The fluid fighters: these can help boost your lymphatic drainage system and help alleviate water retention, which can contribute to cellulite. Try rosemary, sweet fennel, atlas cedarwood, cypress, juniper, grapefruit, geranium or patchouli.

Defining idea...

'Flowers are the sweetest things that God ever made and forgot to put a soul into.'
HENRY WARD BEECHER, US Congregational Minister

*Some essential oils are contraindicated and shouldn't be used during pregnancy or with certain medical conditions so always check with a practitioner.

Here's an idea for you...

Try self-massage. You'll moisturise your cellulitey areas at the same time, making your skin look instantly smoother. Mix six drops of essential oils with 3–4tsp (15–20ml) of carrier oil such as sweet almond, grapeseed or wheatgerm oil. (Don't use essential oils neat on the skin as they can cause irritation.)

The skin enhancers: cellulite looks worse when the skin is dehydrated or as you age and lose that plump firmness of skin. Try rosemary, grapefruit, patchouli, cypress and sweet fennel.

The hormone rebalancers: certain oils are said to help normalise out-of-kilter hormone levels associated with weight gain and cellulite. Try cypress and sweet fennel.

To use the oils either ad to a base oil and rub them in, bathe in them by adding four to six drops to warm water (adding milk or vodka can help disperse the oils), pop them on a tissue and smell them or try burning them in a diffuser and inhaling the scent.

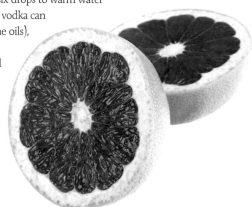

32. The next big thing?

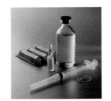

A new treatment has been discovered that could actually destroy fat cells in your cellulite-prone areas – permanently.

The treament involves injecting carbon dioxide directly into the layer of cellulite under the skin to break through cell walls and liquefy the fat, ready for elimination from the body. Carbon dioxide can apparently kill off fat cells in the areas targeted specifically by the injections whilst also widening the capillaries in the skin tissue, resulting in better blood flow and more oxygen and nutrients being delivered to the skin. This may also result in less fluid between the cells, which means firmer skin.

Using a micro-fine needle, the cellulite-sufferer is given several injections, depending on the size of the area being treated, of purified, medically approved carbon dioxide.

Defining idea...

'Any sufficiently advanced technology is indistinguishable from magic.'
ARTHUR C. CLARKE

Here's an idea for you...

Here's an idea for you: The latest thinking on cellulite reduction is to combine two or more salon or medical treatments, rather than sticking to one method. The trick is to choose ones that complement each other so that the end result is to speed up the whole process of diminishing the crinkley stuff. So carbon dioxide therapy, which liquefies fat cells, could be combined with MLD (manual lymphatic drainage) massage, which should help the lymph system expel the mobilised fat cells from your body.

A narrow tube links the needle with a cylinder storing the gas, which in turn is attached to a machine which filters the gas to medical standards and warms it up – cold gas would feel very painful when injected.

Treatments though uncomfortable do not take very long. For the best results, a course of 12–15 treatment sessions is recommended, ideally two per week. One major advantage over other salon treatments is that carbon dioxide therapy has the potential to be long-term.

33. Skin from within

With great nutrition and a little care, you can achieve great-looking skin all over in no time at all.

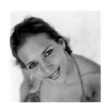

Fruits and vegetables are the main ingredients for a healthy, youthful skin. The reason for this is that they contain lots of vitamins and minerals that perform an antioxidant function, mopping up reactions caused by the free radicals created by such things as stress, pollution and certain foods. Berries and fruits and vegetables with red, purple and blue colouring are particularly good because they're stuffed with antioxidants and contain a group of flavonoids called anthocyanidins, thought to be much more powerful than vitamin E.

Drinking water flushes toxins through your system and hydrates cells carrying essential nutrients to every part of your body. Aim to drink about 2 litres (3.5 pints) daily. Don't overdo it though or you

Here's an idea for you...

Try to eat at least five portions of fruit and vegetables daily. And the more colours the better – try red peppers, yellow peppers, green peppers, red cabbage, sweet potatoes, etc. This way you can get enough antioxidants to help counter the effects of pollution.

could end up flushing minerals out of your system, especially if you're gulping rather than sipping.

Essential fatty acids keep your skin plumped up and moisturised. Do an experiment – take a good quality fish oil supplement for three months (or flax seed if you're vegetarian) and note the quality of skin on the back of your hands. You'll notice that they're better moisturised – and your bum will benefit in the same way. You should also decrease the amount of saturated and processed fats in your diet, as these compete with the good fats and make their job more difficult.

In general, the fresher the food and the more unprocessed it is, the wider the vitamin and mineral range and the more good it will do your skin!

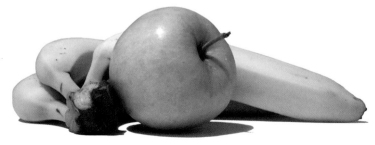

34. Tomorrow's world

Can the latest high-tech laser treatments help zap cellulite away?

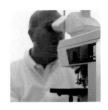

Velasmooth uses a combination of massage rollers and vacuum sucking of the dimply fat (like endermologie) to help break fatty deposits down, and infrared light and radiofrequency (a bit like microwave technoloy). The idea is partly that warming up the fat will soften it and make it easier to disperse. A big plus seems to be that results can be pretty rapid.

Microdermabrasion uses crystals to exfoliate the top layer of skin and reduce the puckering effect. Microdermabrasion cannot make cellulite disappear, but it can make the skin in these areas look and feel a lot smoother and healthier. The treatment can stimulate the production of collagen, which helps prevent cellulite by keeping the fat underneath the skin in place. You can also buy microdermabrasion exfoliators if you fancy trying something similar at home.

Mesotherapy involves a practitioner firing a gun with a micro-fine needle at your cellulite-ridden areas to deliver a tailor-made homeopathic mix of lymphatic drainage and circulation improving plant

Here's an idea for you...

If you're going to invest in a high-tech treatment at a salon, you could try asking the therapist to treat just one buttock or thigh at the first session or two, so you can compare it to the untreated one and see if it's made any difference. It will also give you the chance to see how long the results last once you've left the salon.

extracts, drugs and vitamins into the 'mesoderm', or middle layer of the skin. More modern treatments (called Eporex) use an electrically charged roller to deliver the therapeutic mixture. Can be expensive because you need to go back for top-up treatments.

Endomeso combines endermologie and mesotherapy. You have one session of endermologie on its own, then later the same week you have two back-to-back treatments: endermologie followed by mesotherapy. The idea is that the two therapies complement each other and work better together than they would on their own. This seems very effective for inch loss but less impressive against cellulite and probably the most expensive of all the treatments.

35. Go with the flow

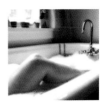

Fluid retention makes cellulite worse, so find out how to beat this problem

Among the causes of water retention are not drinking enough water (the body tries to hang on to the fluid it's got), PMS and too much salt in the diet. Sometimes persistent water retention can mean a health problem more serious than cellulite, so it's a good idea to talk to a health professional to rule this out before starting on a fluid-flushing regime.

Remember not to add salt to food since this will make water retention worse and try these helpful fruits, vegetables and herbs.

Asparagus and avocados are natural diuretics containing potassium, one of the minerals that helps prevent water retention. Spinach and other green leafy vegetables are loaded with magnesium, which helps keep the correct balance of the body's fluids. Broccoli is one of the 'superfoods' that is so packed with nutrients it multi-tasks all over the body, and it contains fluid-busting potassium.

Here's an idea for you...

You can grow parsley easily on your kitchen windowsill so you've always got a handy supply of this fluid-flushing herb. Throw it in soups, sprinkle it on fish dishes, in omelettes, on salads and in sandwiches. When you get it as a garnish in restaurants, don't leave it on the side of your plate – eat it!

Apples are a good source of fluid-flushing potassium and the fibre pectin, which helps keep your system moving. Oranges contain potassium and fibre and so many vitamins you should eat one every day. Grapefruit is good for fibre and potassium and is often used as a detoxifier.

Go for the sweeter pink ones if you're not keen on the acidic taste.

Try drinking herbal teas. Fennel is known as a powerful diuretic and the oil can also help when massaged into your thighs. Parsely is a particularly good diuretic since it contains a chemical called coumarin which helps diminish water retention. Chamomile is a calming herb used for both PMS and water retention. Nettle is highly recommended by herbalists to combat fluid retention and dandelion stimulates urine flow

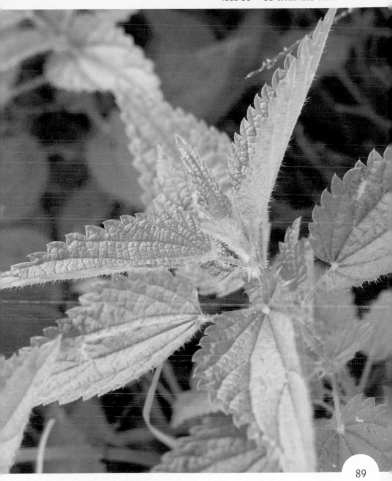

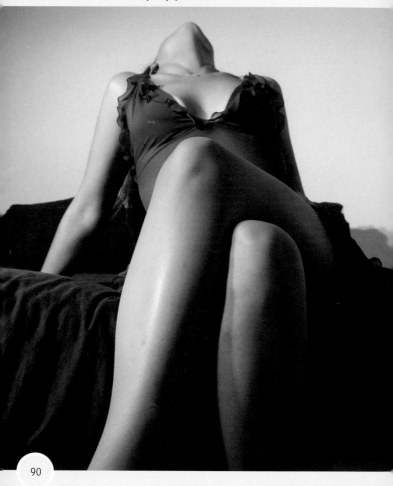

36. The lady vanishes

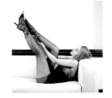

Look inches slimmer with anti-cellulite tights.

Caffeine-impregnated tights sound crazy but could help. Microscopic capsules of gelatine containing caffeine are woven into the tights, and when worn, the heat from the body triggers the breakdown of the capsules, allowing the caffeine to be absorbed through the skin, increasing metabolism and burning fat to reduce cellulite. The caffeine is effective for five washes. They're 20 denier and come in skin tone or black. Buy them on www.palmersshop.com or www.tightsplease.co.uk.

Cellulite-massaging tights massage the skin as you move around, stimulating the skin's microcirculation, easing water retention and reducing cellulite. Some wearers reported less obvious orange-peel skin and reduced thigh circumference after several weeks' wear. They're more expensive than caffeine tights; check out what's available at www.indigohealth.co.uk or www.pantyhose-stockings-hosiery.com.

Compression tights start with a very tight fit at the ankles which gradually lessens as you move up the leg. The graduated compression means the blood circulation is encouraged up the legs and back towards the heart, giving the veinous system a boost – better circulation is supposed to be good for cellulite. These tights could have a cosmetic effect on cellulite-ridden legs by pushing the flesh upwards too, giving you a leg lift while they're on. The compression could have the added effect of squeezing retained fluid up the body and away from the legs, so the legs appear less heavy.

The secret weapon in countless women's underwear drawers are the tights with hold-you-in control pants. These are the tights to go for if you are unlucky enough to have cellulite that can be seen through thin, close-fitting fabrics, such as silky evening skirts or trousers. If you want to smooth out 'saddle-bag' thighs as well, the ones where the reinforced section comes down the thighs a few inches do a great job.

37. Getting into shape

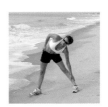

Weight loss is for life and not just for after Christmas.

Newsflash – diets don't work! Permanent weight loss simply means changing your habits, being disciplined and sticking to a healthy eating plan most of the time. Occasionally to avoid the pitfalls of feeling deprived, allow yourself the odd treat.

The trick is to eat foods that will burn slowly and give you sustained energy throughout the day. Ones that burn quickly will rapidly increase your blood sugar levels causing the hormone insulin to be pumped rapidly into the system. The resulting drop in blood sugar will make you feel drowsy. Things that are white and processed burn quickly (white bread, white rice, potatoes, etc.).

Besides lowering the blood sugar, insulin also stores fat, so you may put on weight if your blood sugar is rising and falling like a yo-yo – not good for a shapely behind. You need to be eating foods with plenty of fibre in them (such as vegetables), unprocessed grains, lean protein, essential fats and slow-burning complex carbohydrates. Cutting out stimulants such as tea and coffee in the diet will also help to control the peaks and troughs

Here's an idea for you...

If you're really determined to lose weight, start as you mean to go on and bin unhealthy packages lurking in your cupboards and fridge. Then get hold of the right ingredients: fresh foods and basic dry ingredients like lentils, chickpeas and brown rice.

of blood sugar management. Put simply, don't eat processed foods with highly processed ingredients, which means pretty much anything that comes in a box.

Have a breakfast of porridge with fresh fruit and yoghurt, or eggs on rye toast. For lunch try a great big salad with all the trimmings, but go easy on the dressing – just a little olive oil and lemon juice. End your day with something like grilled fish and broccoli. If you get hungry, a small protein snack will help – nuts and seeds are useful.

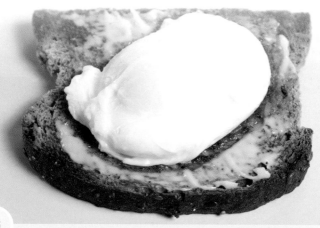

38. Suck it and see

**Liposuction is drastic, but it literally
sucks the fat out of your bottom and
thighs.**

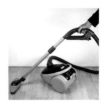

You'll certainly notice a difference after liposuction; bottom and
thighs can measure several inches less and in reducing the amount
of fat the appearance of cellulite is also improved. But it's expensive,
not without risk and discomfort, and cellulite can return if you put
on weight again, since it doesn't tackle the cause of it.

Women who are pear-shaped, so that their bottom half is out of
proportion to the top half, are most likely to benefit from
liposuction to improve cellulite. For these unlucky ladies, no matter
how much they diet and exercise, the bottom-heavy shape will still
remain. Their bodies are simply genetically predisposed to hang on
to fat cells below the waist.

Liposuction is usually performed under a general anaesthetic.
Several small incisions are made to allow a narrow cannula or tube
to access the fat underneath the skin. The fat is then suctioned out

Here's an idea for you...

Get down to your ideal weight before considering liposuction to treat cellulite. As cellulite is a form of fat, if you lose excess weight some of your cellulite will go with it. Once you've got down to your 'fighting weight' you can reassess your cellulite to see if you can deal with the remaining dimples with a less drastic form of treatment.

through the tube. As well as the usual surgical risks, with liposuction, if too much fat and fluid is removed, the body can go into shock and the blood pressure drop drastically, which could be fatal. So make sure you only put your bottom in the hands of an experienced surgeon with an established track record.

Puffiness and swelling post-op will mean that you don't get to see the full benefits of the surgeon's handiwork until your body's had a chance to recover. The holes where the cannulas have been inserted will leave scars, but these should be small and hopefully in places where few people will get the chance to see them.

39. Getting a leg up

Walk your way to firmer, sexier legs with a little help from MBTs, or Masai Barefoot Technology trainers, nicknamed 'fatburners'.

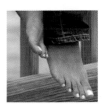

The curved layers of the sole emulate walking on natural, uneven surfaces as opposed to the artificial hard and flat surfaces we mostly walk on today. This forces the body into a more upright posture and means you use muscle groups that are normally neglected. Because the body is working more efficiently and extra muscles are being used, more calories are being burned and weight loss is speeded up. Bottom and leg muscles are toned up more quickly – even while standing the muscles continue working to maintain a centre of balance.

Losing excess fat on bottom and thighs will mean less cellulite. With improved muscle tone over the whole of the lower body, any remaining cellulite will be less visible, and more efficient circulation will boost blood supply to the skin tissues, further improving skin texture.

Defining idea...

'A man's health can be judged by which he takes two at a time – pills or stairs.'
JOAN WELSH

Here's an idea for you...

To get the maximum benefit from wearing MBTs you need to walk as much as you possibly can. So leave the car in the garage and walk to work/to the station/into town/to see friends. Carry your work shoes or evening Manolo Blahniks with you and change when you get there – the longer you wear your MBTs the better the results. The extra exercise will help you lose inches and tone up your bottom even more.

MBTs come in several styles and colours and there's even an open-toed sandal for summer. You can't buy them mail order because they need to be properly fitted to make sure you are using them correctly. They come in slightly more varied sizing than standard footwear and need to fit snugly. The trained fitter will also give you a lesson in how to walk properly in them. For prices and where to buy visit www.mbt-info.com. Roll on!

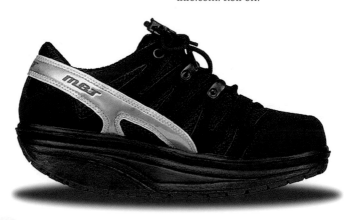

40. Getting your sea legs

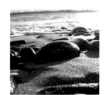

In thalassotherapy mineral-rich seawater feeds the skin and hot and cold water jets stimulate circulation.

The sea contains a virtual A to Z of minerals which can exert beneficial effects on the skin and body. This potent mix includes minerals with antioxidant properties that have a detoxifying and anti-ageing effect. The theory is that through regular soaks in seawater, or warm water with a concentrated mix of sea minerals added, some of these health-giving nutrients are absorbed into the body to help detoxify, diminish water retention, feed the skin and boost its production of new collagen. All of which are big pluses in the battle against cellulite.

In a thalassotherapy treatment alternate hot and cold jets of water are trained on your cellulite. The idea is that the force of the jets coupled with the extremes of temperature crank the circulation up a gear, and sluggish circulation is continually linked to cellulite. The therapist trains the jets at the ankles first and moves up the body so lymph

Here's an idea for you...

Go to the seaside – through there are spas located inland offering treatment, the true definition of a thalassotherapy spa is that it is 300 metres or less from the sea – so you get to spend some therapeutic time on the beach too.

drainage is also encouraged, combating water retention and helping the body rid itself of waste products – two more ways to fight cellulite.

The best spas are found along the French coasts, where you can have jets full of filtered seawater trained on you. Most other countries are not as far advanced with true thalassotherapy using real seawater. Spas in the UK, for instance,

Defining idea...

'The cure for anything is salt water: sweat, tears or the sea.'

ISAK DINESEN, AUTHOR

have not yet made the investment needed to get the seawater piped in, so they may use powdered sea minerals or add seaweed extracts to their baths and pools instead.

41. Out there and doing it

Exercise is great for toning your bum, but if you hate the gym what are the alternatives?

Getting some aerobic exercise by running and walking will obviously increase your cardiovascular fitness, and even in the city (away from busy roads) you'll benefit from breathing 'fresh' air into your lungs. Pumping your heart muscle is important to get your lymph system moving – good for shifting cellulite. So, get out there and do some cardiovascular stuff. Run, jog or walk for at least 20 minutes each day.

In your local park use the benches to stretch, use steps to run up and use lamp posts as distance markers. Let your imagination run wild as to what you can use in the environment to help you in your mission. Set goals – a good one might be to count the number of times you run or walk round the park, each time trying to improve upon the last.

Try power walking – stride out when you walk. Get into it by loading your iPod up with some seriously good music. Skipping is a wonderful way to get your ticker really going and minute for minute

Here's an idea for you...

If getting motivated is a problem try bribing yourself. Put a tick chart on the fridge with your weekly exercise schedule listed, e.g. a run, two walks, step class. Once you've accomplished a month with no passes, allow yourself a treat, such as a massage or new underwear. If you mess up even once during the month, no treat.

burns more calories than jogging. Exercising at home is another way to avoid the gym. Try some squats, lunges, and step ups on your stairs.

Don't forget to stretch at the beginning and end of your workouts. Warm, stretched muscles are muscles that are less likely to be injured.

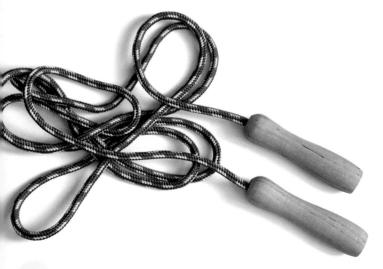

42. Pedal power

Cycling is great exercise for turning a spongy bottom into a pert rear of the year, and for toning and trimming both the back and front of the thighs.

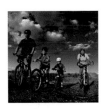

Cycling is a great way to tone up your thigh muscles and gluteus maximus (those big muscles in your bottom). As an aerobic exercise it burns fat and calories and boosts circulation, fighting the build up of cellulite. You don't even have to allow any extra time in your week to fit in this particular cellulite-busting regime – just use it as your primary method of getting from A to B. Before you get in the car to go anywhere, get in the habit of asking yourself, 'Could I get there by bike?'.

There's a newish treatment for cellulite that looks like something out of a spoof sci-fi movie, but could get results. Called Hypoxi-therapy, it combines cycling with vacuum suction. You sit on an

Here's an idea for you...

Don't want to ride alone? Join a cycling club, discover different routes to ride and open up a whole new, fun side to your social life. And there will always be someone around to help you mend that puncture.

exercise bike and pedal away, but from the waist down you are enclosed in a futuristic 'slimming pod' vacuum chamber. While your pedal power burns the calories, the vacuum's sucking action increases the blood supply to your below-the-belt cellulitey areas, accelerating fat and cellulite breakdown.

This does take a bit of effort – one tester described it as similar to cycling through sand – and money (around £450 for a course of a dozen 30-minute sessions over a period of a month), but there have been some satisfied customers. One woman lost half a stone and about 45% of her cellulite. Find out more at www.hypoxitraining.com.

43. Ladykillers

The higher your levels of the female hormone oestrogen the more likely you are to have cellulite.

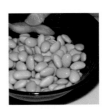

Oestrogen is linked to fat and the way it is stored in the body. If women put on weight their bodies produce more oestrogen, and those with high levels of oestrogen tend to have extra fat around their bottom, hips and thighs. Oestrogen also encourages fluid retention, which some experts believe is key to causing cellulite.

We can't really control how much oestrogen we've got or where our body stores fat, but we can give it less fat to store. There is no need to buy any special 'diet' foods, or follow specific diet regimes unless you want to. Simple strategies such as cutting down on the obvious high-fat foods such as cheese, butter, full-fat milk, (make sure you're getting your protein and calcium elsewhere) bacon, burgers

Here's an idea for you...

American cellulite and weight loss expert Dr Sandra Cabot says pear-shaped women should include as many phytoestrogen-containing foods as possible in their diet, since these have a balancing effect on the oestrogen-dependent fatty deposits. Soya and soya-based products and linseeds are high in phytoestrogens.

Defining idea...

'You have breasts and you have cellulite. Now you are a real woman.'
Paris-based beautician to transexual clients undergoing hormone treatment

and processed foods and piling on the fruit and vegetables and cooking from scratch can make a big difference. Beware of buying low-fat versions of foods, such as yoghurts – these often have lower fat but more sugar, which won't do your cellulite any good either.

If you're a high oestrogen, pear-shaped kind of girl, get those legs moving with speed-walking, cycling or running to both burn off fat quickly and tone the whole of your lower body. If you've got a big bottom, this will help turn it from a wobbly blancmange into a high, sexy firm globe.

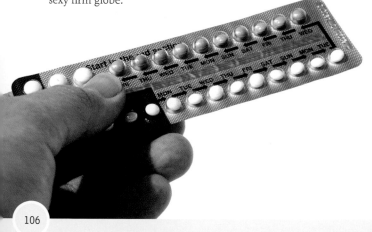

44. Waste disposal

Follow short-term detox cleansing regimes to help the liver get rid of waste products – including those that could increase cellulite.

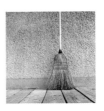

Experts are unsure how central a role toxin build up plays in the problem of cellulite. It's certainly true that the body has its own natural detoxifier – the liver – which will break down harmful substances from food, drink or other sources. But why not give it a helping hand?

Try a simple, calming and restorative detox strategy of between two and five days. Back up dietary adjustments with body care and anti-cellulite strategies such as dry skin brushing, massage, exfoliation and moisturising to give your skin a healthy glow.

■ Ditch the alcohol and caffeine and drink only water (at least 6 glasses per day), herbal teas or fresh fruit and vegetable juices.

Defining idea...

'Nothing in excess.'
Inscription on the temple of Apollo at Delphi

Here's an idea for you...

Freshly liquidised fruit and vegetable juices and smoothies are especially good for detoxing because the less energy your body needs to digest food, the more it will have to cleanse your system of toxins. Fresh juices are also an easy way of making sure you get your five portions of fruit and veg a day.

- Ban sugar, chocolate, saturated animal fats (e.g. butter), processed foods and ready meals.
- Avoid adding salt to the food you cook.
- Eat plenty of fruit and vegetables, organic and raw if possible, as salads, crudites or plates of cut fruit.
- Include bananas because they are filling, potassium-rich (good for balancing the body's fluid levels), great energy boosters and full of fibre.
- Avoid red meat, getting high-quality protein from nuts, pulses, wholegrains, fresh fish and organic chicken and eggs.
- Try to avoid stress, especially if you're the sort of girl who wants to comfort eat when she's under pressure.
- Walk, run or cycle in fresh air – get as far away from pollution as you can.
- Go to bed early and get lots of restorative sleep.

45. Take a walk on the wild side

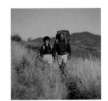

Stay in peak condition and keep your legs and bum in trim whilst at the same time gaining a bit of perspective on life.

Walking means more than popping out to the corner shop for twenty Marlboro. Get out into the countryside and try some real walking. Just make sure you're kitted out with the right gear before you set out:

- Waterproofs – these days you can get very light wet-weather gear that will fold up and fit into you pocket. Don't just get the top, invest in the trousers as well – there's nothing worse than being in the middle of nowhere with wet, cold trousers and no chance of changing them for the next 50 miles.

- The second vital bit of kit for your proper walking experience is the right boots and proper walking socks. A good outdoor shop should be able to advise on the right kind of boots and socks for you. The boots need to be protective of the ankles, waterproof and not too heavy. They also need a good grip – the proper lace-up ones are ideal.

Here's an idea for you...

Start small. Going on long walks can seem quite scary if you're new to them and can't read a map, but the gear is only necessary if you're going to take the whole thing seriously – short walks in the countryside on designated footpaths don't need full-on survival gear. Always take water with you, however!

- Choose a rucksack with a middle strap that goes round your tummy as this will help to protect your back. These days there are rucksacks that make sure that the material isn't next to your back so you don't get too sweaty carrying it. Make sure you get one with pockets for maps, bottles of water, etc.

- Water, sunscreen, a hat, plasters (for blisters) and a reliable map should all go in your rucksack.

46. Dance with a stranger

Joining a dance class could help us drop a dress size, while having fun and learning something new.

Ballet for grown-ups. If you have cellulite or wobbly bits on your inner thighs, ballet is the dance for you. Just standing in a basic ballet position with your heels together and toes apart at 45 degrees starts to work the backs of the legs and thighs. Moves such as the arabesque, when you lift a leg up at an angle that really squeezes the gluteus maximus, are just what a wobbly bottom needs. If you practice the moves at home too you should start to notice a subtle change in your body shape within just a few weeks.

Sexy salsa. With all that twisting and turning, stomping and leg kicking, salsa really works the bottom, legs, waist and hips. There's now such a huge enthusiasm for salsa that you shouldn't have too

Here's an idea for you...

If you're single, make sure you choose a class where you have to dance with a partner. It takes two to tango, waltz or ballroom, and meeting someone new will give you an added incentive to dance your cellulite away – before he gets a chance to see it.

much trouble finding a class, and no, you don't have to bring a dance partner, swapping partners is part of the fun.

Street dance. This is the kind of dance you see in pop videos and commercials and classes can be a mix of different styles – hip-hop, jazz, anything goes as long as it's funky, lively and fun. These are some of the most aerobic dance classes there are (talk to the teacher about your fitness level first before signing up), and aerobic dance is one of the fastest ways to lose excess baggage around the hips and thighs. It gives the circulation a sure-fire boost as well as the metabolism, which helps in the battle against cellulite.

47. Bend it, stretch it

Follow the deep-stretching technique pioneered by movement and dance expert Marja Putkisto, to boost circulation and lymph drainage in the legs and smooth out cellulite.

Try these stretches to improve cellulite four or five times a week. To get maximum benefit, make sure you eat healthily, drink plenty of water and walk 20 minutes a day.

Lizard stretch to lengthen muscles around hips and pelvis

- Kneel on the floor, bend the right leg to create a 90-degree angle in front of your body with the foot flat on the floor.
- Extend your back leg behind you, staying upright with your chest lifted, and tilt your tailbone towards your navel.
- Rotate your back leg from your hip joint slightly inwards.
- Breathe in through the nose, focusing on the air reaching the lowest part of the lungs, then exhale slowly through your mouth, creating the stretch at the end of the outbreath.

Here's an idea for you...

Breathing deeply, so the air reaches the bottom of your lungs and not just the top, and slow, deep stretches that you hold for a couple of minutes have a brilliant de-stressing effect when you do them together. You may even become so laid back that you'll stop worrying about your cellulite altogether.

- Continue the stretch with the flow of your breathing, applying more body weight through your pelvis to increase the stretch, for two to five minutes.
- Repeat on the other side.

Fishtail stretch for pelvis and thighs

- Lie on the floor on your right side and support your head with your right arm.
- Turn your tailbone slightly towards your navel.
- Straighten your right leg. Bend your left knee and place your left foot on the floor in front of your right knee.
- Place your left hand on the floor.
- Inhale deeply through your nose, press your left hand into the floor, squeeze your sitting bones closer to each other and lift your waistline off the floor.
- Exhale, pause, and lift the right leg about 10cm off the floor.
- Keep breathing deeply and slowly and focus on the inner thigh muscles, holding the stretch for two minutes or longer if possible.
- Repeat on the other side.

48. Some like it hot

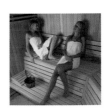

Saunas and steam rooms open up sweat pores and may help eliminate cellulite-causing toxins

Too much of the stress hormone cortisol can set off a chain of reactions in the body which could have detrimental effects on the digestion and skin, and even lead to weight gain – none of which is going to do your cellulite any good. But the de-stressing benefits of a sauna can last long after you've put your clothes back on

The perfect time to head for the sauna or steam room is after some anti-cellulite exercise – you'll get the extra benefit of the heat acting as a muscle relaxant, which will help ease any post-workout soreness or stiffness. Your body will start to react to the sauna heat as soon as you step through the door. The temperature makes the heart rate increase, so the circulation is boosted. Improved circulation is good for cellulite-prone skin, and it also gives the body's waste disposal system a shove in the right direction,

Defining idea...

'Every time a woman leaves off something she looks better, but every time a man leaves off something he looks worse.'
WILL ROGERS

helping to speed up the rate at which toxins are expelled. The heat also opens up the skin's pores, which may further encourage the elimination of toxins.

Because the pores have been opened up and cleansed, post-sauna could also be a good time to massage any anti-cellulite creams into your dimples. Take your lotions and potions with you so you can slather them on before you get dressed.

Extreme temperatures in any type of sauna have a dramatic impact on your body so be sure to read the health warning notices outside the sauna door, and don't be tempted to stay longer than the recommended time, however de-stressing it is in there.

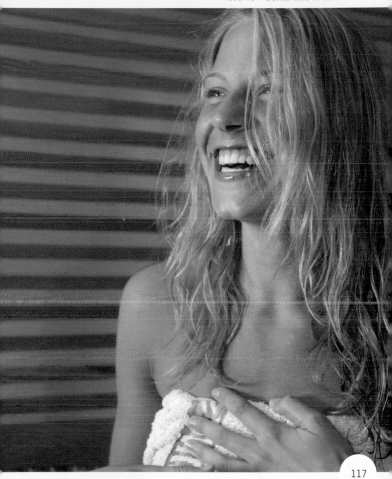

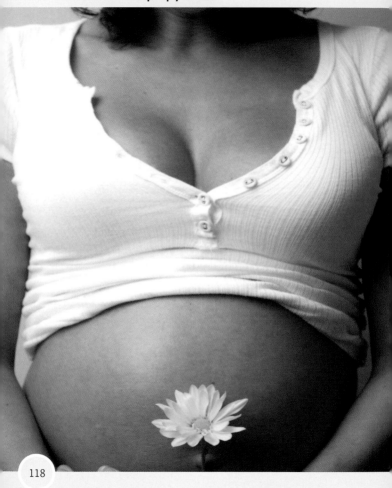

49. Mums, bums and tums

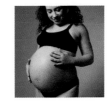

**Extra pounds and hormonal surges during pregnancy often make cellulite worse.
Here's how to avoid surplus weight and firm up after your baby's born.**

It's completely normal to take six months or more to shift the extra weight, and because of weight gain and increased oestrogen levels it's also completely normal for cellulite to increase during pregnancy and to still be there afterwards.

Cellulite gained in pregnancy doesn't have to be permanent though, and there are ways you can have a healthy pregnancy and minimise the amount of orange peel you're going to get. You need sufficient calories, but it's important to eat nutrient-rich foods including lots of fruits and

Here's an idea for you.

Many new mothers find the weight drops off quickly if they carry on breastfeeding for as long as they can because of the hefty amount of calories breastfeeding uses up. With weight loss goes cellulite loss, and the baby gets the best nutrition possible from your milk – so everyone wins.

vegetables and try to ditch any junk food habits and sugary stuff – just the sort of diet that's anti-cellulite, in fact. The amount of weight you should gain over the whole nine months is between 25lb and 35lb. After the first three months, putting on an average of one pound a week is about right.

If you carry on with regular but gentle exercise throughout your pregnancy you'll also help keep cellulite at bay. You can walk or swim right up to the end, or try one of the classes specially designed for pregnant women.

Be careful about exercising apart from taking your baby out for a walk for the first few weeks after the birth and check with your doctor or midwife before you start any exercise to make sure you're ready, particularly if you've had any complications or a Caesarean. If you're breastfeeding, it's a good idea to exercise straight afterwards so your breasts won't be painfully full of milk and your baby is likely to be asleep.

50. Grass roots

Clinical trials show that the herb gotu kola could improve cellulite.

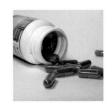

Studies suggest the herb's abilities include stimulating the body's production of substances that strengthen the connective tissues that keep the fat cells in place. Gotu kola can improve circulation and blood flow, which is why it has been used for centuries to help heal skin diseases and treat varicose veins and other problems caused by reduced blood flow. Still more studies show that it could help by stimulating the lymph system to get rid of excess fluids – the dreaded water retention that makes cellulite look worse.

Gotu kola is one of very few herbs that has been investigated with a clinical trial specifically for its effect on cellulite. In a study of 65 women carried out over a three month period seventy-eight per cent noticed a difference in their cellulite.

Here's an idea for you...

As with so many cellulite-shifting methods, think of this herb as part of an overall plan of attack rather than a solo solution. Taking gotu kola but sticking to a zero-exercise and junk food regime will just be money down the drain.

Defining idea...

'The method of nature: who could ever analyse it?'
RALPH WALDO EMERSON

You can find gotu kola in supplement form in pharmacies and health food stores. Herbalists reckon 30mg three times a day is sufficient to strengthen the connective tissue and keep skin smooth. The dried herb can be used to make a tea which you can drink several times a day. You can buy it from health shops and herbalists who will be able to give you advice on how much to use. Buy gotu kola in tincture form and squeeze a few drops into a little water. Oil and creams containing gotu kola can be used to massage into the body to rehydrate the skin.*

*Some essential oils are contraindicated and shouldn't be used during pregnancy or with certain medical conditions so always check with a practitioner.

51. The winds of change

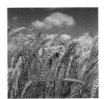

Bloating's not the only side-effect of wheat intolerance; it may also make cellulite worse.

If you are wheat intolerant your absorption of vitamins and minerals may be inhibited, toxin elimination may be less efficiant and bloating caused by excess gas in the system – from food that hasn't been broken down properly – may be impairing the lymph system. All problems linked to cellulite.

Trouble is, so much of the western diet is based on wheat and this, according to some nutritionists, is part of the problem. Mass produced wheat is relatively cheap and it is used in countless manufactured foods, turning up in unexpected places from ready-to-cook dinners to sauces, salad dressings, crisps and other snacks.

The good news is that there are ever-increasing options for the wheat avoider and the bigger supermarkets will have whole sections of wheat-free goodies. Many wheat-sensitive people find once they have cut back and reduced or eliminated their uncomfortable symptoms, they can reintroduce small amounts of wheat to their diet.

Here's an idea for you...

According to dieticians, the first thing to do if you are experiencing discomfort after eating certain foods is to keep a food diary for two weeks and write down everything you eat and any symptoms. The first person to show this to is your GP, who will decide whether to refer you to a dietician for further investigation.

- Replace bread with oatcakes, rice cakes, Ryvita, taco shells or wheat-free breads.
- For breakfast try switching to corn or rice-based cereals such as corn flakes, porridge and wheat-free muesli. Alternatively start the day with yogurt and fruit.
- Salad and soup is a good swap at lunchtime instead of sandwiches or try rice-based sushi.
- Replace regular pasta with pasta made from rice or corn, or choose rice or rice noodles instead.
- Reach for the fruit bowl instead of the biscuit tin or if you really can't hack it without something gooey, go for oatcakes with low-sugar jam. Wheat-free biscuits are available – but remember sugar-laden biscuits of any type are best avoided if you're serious about getting rid of cellulite.

52. Getting plastered

Cellulite-busting patches that you stick on your bottom and thighs send skin-improving minerals to your trouble spots.

Like nicotine patches, the ingredients in an anti-cellulite patch are designed to be slowly absorbed into the skin over a certain period. A peel-off adhesive strip allows you to stick them on your worst-offending areas, then you just leave them there to do their job, while you carry on and do whatever you want.

Some look very small but the theory is that the ingredients spread outwards to treat an area several times bigger than the patch itself – which may be a relief for those of us with family-sized crinkley bottoms. One of the main ingredients in the patches is caffeine. Other ingredients usually include mineral, herbal or seaweed algae extracts aimed at either draining fluid from the tissues in the area, boosting the skin's microcirculation or improving skin

Here's an idea for you...

Don't be tempted to think that because caffeine is being used in a patch to combat cellulite that it must be alright to drink it. It's still better from a detox point of view to drink herbal tea instead. Sorry.

Defining idea...

'Taking joy in living is a woman's best cosmetic.'
ROSALIND RUSSELL

texture. Many of the ingredients are similar to the ones in anti-cellulite creams – the idea is that they are absorbed by the skin more easily via patches. Ingredients may be activated by body heat, which apparently aids absorption.

The experiences of women trying patches vary widely, from 'couldn't see any difference' to the loss of as much as 4cm from their thigh circumference and smoother looking skin after wearing the patches for a month. The patches worked best when teamed with other anti-cellulite ideas. It may be that, like some of the creams, the role of patches is to improve the appearance of the skin over the cellulite – so that it looks firmer and smoother – rather than affect the underlying cellulite itself.

As with any product, it's safer to buy from established brand names than those you've never heard of, and always follow manufacturers' instructions to the letter.

This book is published by Infinite Ideas, creators of the acclaimed **52 Brilliant Ideas series**. If you found this book helpful, there are other titles in the **Brilliant Little Ideas** series which you may also find of interest.

- **Be incredibly creative:** 52 brilliant little ideas to hone your mind
- **Catwalk looks:** 52 brilliant little ideas to look gorgeous always
- **Drop a dress size:** 52 brilliant little ideas to lose weight and stay slim
- **Find your dream job:** 52 brilliant little ideas for total career happiness
- **Heal your troubled mind:** 52 brilliant little ideas for defeating depression
- **Healthy children's lunches:** 52 brilliant little ideas for junk-free meals kids will love
- **Incredible sex:** 52 brilliant little ideas to take you all the way
- **Make your money work:** 52 brilliant little ideas for rescuing your finances
- **Perfect romance:** 52 brilliant little ideas for finding and keeping a lover
- **Raising young children:** 52 brilliant little ideas for parenting under 5s
- **Relax:** 52 brilliant little ideas to chill out
- **Shape up your bum:** 52 brilliant little ideas for maximising your gluteus

For more detailed information on these books and others published by Infinite Ideas please visit www.infideas.com.

See reverse for order form.

Qty	Title	RRP
	Be incredibly creative	£5.99
	Catwalk looks	£5.99
	Drop a dress size	£5.99
	Find your dream job	£5.99
	Heal your troubled mind	£5.99
	Healthy children's lunches	£5.99
	Incredible sex	£5.99
	Make your money work	£5.99
	Perfect romance	£5.99
	Raising young children	£5.99
	Relax	£5.99
	Shape up your bum	£5.99

Add £2.49 postage per delivery address

Final TOTAL

Name: ....

Delivery address: ....

....

....

E-mail:................................Tel (in case of problems): ....

By post Fill in all relevant details, cut out or copy this page and send along with a cheque made payable to Infinite Ideas. Send to: *Brilliant Little Ideas*, Infinite Ideas, 36 St Giles, Oxford OX1 3LD. **Credit card orders over the telephone** Call +44 (0) 1865 514 888. Lines are open 9am to 5pm Monday to Friday.

Please note that no payment will be processed until your order has been dispatched. Goods are dispatched through Royal Mail within 14 working days, when in stock. We never forward personal details on to third parties or bombard you with junk mail. The prices quoted are for UK and RoI residents only. If you are outside these areas please contact us for postage and packing rates. Any questions or comments please contact us on 01865 514 888 or email info@infideas.com.